# Alternative healing: Cancer treatment and other common illnesses

# Table of contents

# Quotes on alternative medicine and healing

"Eat your food as your medicine. Otherwise you have to eat medicine as your food." ~ Steve Jobs

Herbs are the friend of the physician and the pride of cooks." ~ Charlemagne.

"All that man needs for health and healing has been provided by God in nature, the Challenge of science is to find it." ~ Paracelsus.

"There are no incurable diseases — only the lack of will. There are no worthless herbs — only the lack of knowledge." ~ Avicenna

# Introduction

Welcome to a one-of-a-kind book that takes an unconventional alternative to achieving optimal health! While conventional medicine has its advantages, the purpose of this guide is to introduce you to the incredible advantages of natural therapy and healing formulas. You'll learn how to take a holistic and personalized approach to supporting your overall well-being and addressing common health issues like cancer. Prepare to discover a world of possibilities and unleash nature's power to transform your life!

# Chapter One

## Introduction to herbs that can assist in the treatment of cancer plus others

While some herbs have shown promise in laboratory studies, it is important to note that there is currently no definitive evidence that any specific herb can cure cancer. Herbal remedies should not be used as a substitute for proven medical treatments such as chemotherapy, radiation, and surgery.

However, these alternative medicines could be immensely helpful to prevent and minimize cancerous cells from ravaging and destroying our body system, and in the long run make us healthier.

That being said, here are some herbs that have been studied for their potential anti-cancer properties:

- Turmeric: Curcumin, the active ingredient in turmeric, has been shown to have anti-inflammatory and anti-cancer properties in laboratory studies.

Turmeric's medicinal health benefits

Turmeric, also known as Curcuma longa, is a plant that belongs to the ginger family. It is a popular spice commonly used in Asian cuisine, particularly in Indian, Pakistani, and Bangladeshi dishes. Turmeric is known for its distinct yellow color, which comes from the compound curcumin.

In traditional medicine, turmeric has been used for its medicinal properties for thousands of years. It is considered a natural anti-inflammatory and antioxidant, and its active ingredient, curcumin, has been studied extensively for its potential health benefits. Here are some of the potential health benefits of turmeric:

Anti-inflammatory properties: Turmeric has anti-inflammatory properties and has been used to alleviate pain and inflammation associated with arthritis and other inflammatory conditions.

Antioxidant properties: Curcumin, the active ingredient in turmeric, has antioxidant properties that help protect the body from damage caused by free radicals.

Digestive health: Turmeric has been used to improve digestion and reduce symptoms of digestive disorders such as bloating and gas.

Brain health: Studies suggest that curcumin may have a protective effect on the brain and may help prevent or reduce the risk of neurodegenerative diseases such as Alzheimer's and Parkinson's disease.

Heart health: Curcumin has been shown to improve heart health by reducing inflammation and oxidative stress.

Turmeric can be consumed in various forms, including as a spice in cooking, in supplement form, or as a tea. However, it is important to note that the active ingredient in turmeric, curcumin, is not easily absorbed by the body. Therefore, supplements that contain piperine (a compound found in black pepper) or a form of curcumin that is more easily absorbed by the body may be more effective. As with any supplement or medicinal herb, it is important to consult with a healthcare professional before use.

- Garlic: Several studies have suggested that garlic may have anti-cancer properties, particularly against stomach and colorectal cancers.

Garlic Medicinal Health Benefits

Garlic (Allium ) is a plant in the onion family that is widely used as a flavoring in food. It has also been used for its medicinal properties for thousands of years. Garlic contains several compounds that have been found to have health benefits, including allicin, ajoene, and alliin.

Some of the potential health benefits of garlic include:

Lowering blood pressure: Garlic has been shown to have a modest effect on reducing blood pressure in people with high blood pressure.

Reducing cholesterol levels: Garlic can help reduce total cholesterol and LDL ("bad") cholesterol levels in the blood, which may help prevent heart disease.

Boosting immune function: Garlic has antimicrobial properties and may help boost the immune system, potentially reducing the risk of infections.

Preventing blood clots: Garlic has blood-thinning properties that may help prevent the formation of blood clots, which can cause heart attacks and strokes.

Fighting cancer: Some studies suggest that garlic may have cancer-fighting properties, although more research is needed in this area.

Garlic is generally considered safe for most people when consumed in food amounts. However, taking garlic supplements or large amounts of garlic can cause side effects such as bad breath, body odor, and digestive problems. I recommend that you take it more at night(especially to bed), with plenty of water. It may also interact with certain medications, so it is important to talk to a healthcare provider before taking garlic supplements if you are on medication.

Conclusively,  garlic is a tasty and healthy addition to your diet, and may have a number of potential health benefits.

- Ginger: Ginger has been shown to have anti-inflammatory and anti-cancer properties, and may also help to reduce nausea and vomiting during cancer treatment.

Ginger's Medicinal Health Benefits

Ginger is a root that has been used for centuries in traditional medicine to treat a variety of ailments. Here are some of the medicinal health benefits associated with ginger:

Anti-inflammatory properties: Ginger has powerful anti-inflammatory properties that can help alleviate pain and swelling associated with conditions such as osteoarthritis, rheumatoid arthritis, and other inflammatory conditions.

Nausea relief: Ginger has been shown to be effective in reducing nausea and vomiting, particularly in cases of morning sickness, motion sickness, and post-operative nausea.

Digestive aid: Ginger can help stimulate digestion, relieve bloating, and reduce gas. It has also been used to treat stomach ulcers and other digestive issues.

Immune system booster: Ginger has high levels of antioxidants and other compounds that can help boost the immune system and protect against illnesses.

Heart health: Some research has suggested that ginger can help lower cholesterol levels and improve heart health by reducing the risk of heart disease.

Pain relief: Ginger has been shown to be effective in reducing pain associated with menstrual cramps, headaches, and muscle soreness.

Nonetheless, ginger is a versatile and powerful herb that can provide numerous health benefits. However, it's important to consult with a healthcare professional before using ginger as a treatment for any medical condition.

- Onions: This spice is very useful in building our immune system and assisting in the fight against cancerous growth.

Onions' medicinal  health benefits

Onions are a popular vegetable that are used in cooking all over the world, but they also have a number of potential medicinal health benefits. Here are a few:

Anti-inflammatory properties: Onions contain compounds such as quercetin and sulfur, which have been shown to have anti-inflammatory effects. This can be helpful in reducing inflammation in the body, which is associated with a range of health problems.

Immune-boosting: Onions are rich in vitamin C, which is an important nutrient for supporting immune function. They also contain other nutrients like zinc and selenium, which are known to have immune-boosting properties.

Heart health: Onions contain flavonoids that have been shown to help lower blood pressure and reduce the risk of heart disease. They can also help improve cholesterol levels by lowering LDL ("bad") cholesterol.

Cancer prevention: Some studies have suggested that the compounds found in onions, particularly sulfur compounds, may have anti-cancer properties. For example, they may help prevent the growth and spread of certain types of cancer cells.

Digestive health: Onions contain a type of fiber called inulin, which can help promote the growth of beneficial gut bacteria. This can have a positive effect on digestive health, as well as overall health and well-being.

It's worth noting that while onions may have these potential health benefits, they are not a substitute for medical treatment or a healthy lifestyle. If you have a health condition, it's important to talk to your healthcare provider about the best course of treatment.

- Green tea: The polyphenols in green tea have been shown to have anti-cancer properties in laboratory studies, although the evidence is mixed when it comes to human studies.

Green Tea and it's medicinal health benefits

Green tea is a type of tea made from the leaves of the Camellia  plant. It has been used for centuries in traditional medicine, and modern research has confirmed that it offers a variety of medicinal health benefits. Here are some of the potential health benefits of drinking green tea:

Antioxidant properties: Green tea is rich in antioxidants called polyphenols, which can help protect your body from damage caused by free radicals.

Reduced risk of cardiovascular disease: Studies have shown that drinking green tea can help lower blood pressure and reduce the risk of cardiovascular disease.

Weight management: Green tea may help boost metabolism and increase fat burning, which can aid in weight loss.

Reduced risk of cancer: The antioxidants in green tea may help prevent the development and growth of cancer cells.

Improved brain function: Green tea contains caffeine, which can help improve brain function, as well as an amino acid called L-theanine, which can promote relaxation and reduce anxiety.

Improved dental health: The catechins in green tea can help kill bacteria in the mouth, which can improve dental health and reduce the risk of cavities and bad breath.

Reduced risk of type 2 diabetes: Green tea may help regulate blood sugar levels and reduce the risk of developing type 2 diabetes.

Reduced inflammation: The polyphenols in green tea have anti-inflammatory properties, which can help reduce inflammation in the body and improve overall health.

In a nutshell, drinking green tea can be a simple and enjoyable way to incorporate healthy habits into your daily routine. However, it's important to keep in mind that green tea should not be used as a substitute for medical treatment, and you should talk to your doctor before making any significant changes to your diet or health routine.

- Milk thistle: Milk thistle has been shown to have anti-inflammatory and antioxidant properties, and some studies suggest that it may have a protective effect against certain types of cancer.

Milk Thistle General Health Benefits.

Milk thistle (Silybum marianum) is a plant that has been used for medicinal purposes for thousands of years. It is a member of the daisy family and is native to the Mediterranean region. The plant has distinctive purple flowers and large, spiky leaves with white veins.

Milk thistle is known for its medicinal properties, particularly in its ability to support liver health. The active ingredient in milk thistle is a flavonoid called silymarin, which is a powerful antioxidant that can help protect liver cells from damage. It is also thought to help improve liver function and reduce inflammation.

In addition to its liver-protective properties, milk thistle has been used to treat a variety of other conditions, including:

Digestive disorders: Milk thistle has been used to treat digestive issues such as bloating, constipation, and indigestion.

High cholesterol: Some studies have found that milk thistle can help lower cholesterol levels, which may be beneficial for people with high cholesterol.

Type 2 diabetes: Milk thistle may help improve insulin resistance and blood sugar levels in people with type 2 diabetes.

Skin conditions: Some research suggests that milk thistle may help improve certain skin conditions, such as psoriasis.

Milk thistle is available in various forms, including capsules, extracts, and teas. It is generally considered safe for most people, but it can cause mild side effects such as diarrhea, nausea, and bloating in some individuals. As with any herbal supplement, it is important to talk to your healthcare provider before using milk thistle to make sure it is safe for you and does not interfere with any medications you may be taking.

- Cloves: Cloves are an aromatic spice that is widely used in cooking and traditional medicine. They are the dried flower buds of the Syzygium tree, which is native to the Maluku Islands in Indonesia.

Cloves are small, dark brown, and have a tapered, nail-like shape. They have a strong, pungent flavor and aroma, with a warm, sweet, and slightly bitter taste. Cloves contain a high concentration of essential oils, especially eugenol, which gives them their distinctive scent and flavor.

In cooking, cloves are used as a flavoring agent in many sweet and savory dishes. They are commonly used in spice blends, such as pumpkin pie spice and garam masala, and are also used to flavor meats, stews, soups, and sauces.

Cloves have also been used for centuries in traditional medicine for their various health benefits. They have antimicrobial and anti-inflammatory properties and have been used to treat toothaches, digestive issues, respiratory problems, and other ailments.

In all facets, cloves are a versatile spice with a unique flavor and aroma that can add depth and complexity to many different dishes.

It is important to consult with a healthcare professional before taking any herbal remedies, as they can interact with other medications and have potential side effects.

# Chapter Two

## Secret nuggets to support the treatment and prevention of cancer plus others via herbs.

### Nugget One

Carefully grate the cloves, onions, garlic, ginger and turmeric etc into paste form.

Put inside a jar or container with a cover and pour warm water to soak it up for at least one hour. You can also add pure honey to it, if you deem fit.

Mix the mixture together and scoop with a spoon( for as much as you can) every six to eight hours in a day (24hours).

Note: Prepare what you can consume for a day (24 hours) and make sure you consume it for that day for effective results.

If this is done for about three times a week continually, there will be noticeable positive changes to that ill health condition.

***Remember that this is not only for cancer problems but other common and related health conditions like kidney problems, liver issues, blood sugar levels and immune system booster, to mention but a few.***

**Nugget Two**

Take some quantities of these medicinal spices. ( Ginger, garlic, turmeric, cloves, onions etc)

Break the spice into small pieces or bits or rather cut into small pieces or bits. Boil them together and add one or two bags of green tea to it, allow it to simmer for about 10 minutes.

Allow it to steep  and cool down for another 10 minutes then, sieve out the water and drink it warm.

Do this first thing in the morning and last thing at night preferably on an empty stomach.

Make it a routine and a lifestyle.

You will notice substantial positive changes to your ill health condition.

***Remember that it is not only for cancer problems but other common and related health issues.***

*Note*: Take as much quantity of each of the spices, as you deem okay. However, start with small quantities and observe the result before increasing  them. All the same,  let the quantity of each of  the spices  used together be virtually the same.

## Cancer-fighting Leaves

There are several plants and their leaves that are known for their potential anti-cancer properties. However, it is important to note that none of these plants or leaves should be used as a replacement for medical treatment, and any use should be discussed with a healthcare professional.

Here are a few examples of leaves that are thought to have anti-cancer properties:

- Green tea leaves and Benefits

Green tea is known for its antioxidant and anti-inflammatory properties, which may help prevent cancer cell growth.

Green tea leaves are derived from the Camellia plant, which is native to China and other parts of Asia. It has been consumed for thousands of years and is known for its many health benefits.

One of the main benefits of green tea leaves is that they are rich in antioxidants, which can help to protect the body against damage caused by free radicals. This can help to reduce the risk of a variety of diseases, including cancer, heart disease, and Alzheimer's disease.

Green tea leaves also contain a number of other beneficial compounds, including caffeine, L-theanine, and catechins.

- Turmeric leaves and Benefits

Turmeric contains a compound called curcumin, which has been found to have anti-cancer properties in some studies.
Turmeric leaves are the leaves of the turmeric plant, which is a popular spice

used in many culinary dishes and traditional medicines, it also has anti-inflammatory properties.

- Moringa leaves and Benefits

Moringa is a plant that has been used for centuries in traditional medicine. It contains compounds that have been shown to have anti-cancer properties.

Moringa leaves are highly nutritious and have been traditionally used in many cultures for their medicinal properties. Some of the potential benefits of consuming Moringa leaves include:

Rich in nutrients: Moringa leaves are a good source of vitamins, minerals, and antioxidants, including vitamin C, vitamin A, calcium, potassium, and iron.

Boosts Immunity: Moringa leaves contain high levels of vitamin C and other antioxidants that can help strengthen the immune system and fight off infections.

Reduces inflammation: Moringa leaves contain anti-inflammatory compounds that can help reduce inflammation in the body, which is a contributing factor to many chronic diseases.

Lowers blood sugar: Moringa leaves have been shown to lower blood sugar levels in people with diabetes, likely due to their high fiber content and ability to improve insulin sensitivity.

- Wheatgrass leaves and Benefits

Wheatgrass is a popular superfood that is known for its high nutrient content. Some studies suggest that wheatgrass may have anti-cancer properties.

Wheatgrass is a type of young grass that is harvested from the wheat plant Triticum . It is packed with nutrients, including vitamins, minerals, amino acids, and antioxidants, and has been used for its health benefits for centuries. Some potential benefits of consuming wheatgrass:

Wheatgrass is rich in nutrients like vitamins A, C, and E, as well as iron, magnesium, calcium, and amino acids.

- Dandelion leaves and Benefits

Dandelion is a plant that is often used in traditional medicine to treat various ailments. Some studies have found that dandelion may have anti-cancer properties and it can be eaten either crooked or raw.

Dandelion leaves benefits are summarily listed below:

It promotes liver health.

Boost  immune system

Reduces cancer risk

Lowers blood pressure

Reduces inflammation

Regulating blood sugar and cholesterol

Providing antioxidants

- Pawpaw leaves and Benefits

Pawpaw leaves have been traditionally used for their medicinal properties, and recent studies have shown that they contain various bioactive compounds that can provide numerous health benefits. Some of the potential medicinal benefits of pawpaw leaves include:

Boosting the immune system: Pawpaw leaves are rich in antioxidants, which help to boost the immune system and protect the body against oxidative stress.

Treating malaria: Pawpaw leaves contain alkaloids such as carpaine, which has been found to have antimalarial properties.

Lowering blood sugar levels: Some studies suggest that pawpaw leaves can help regulate blood sugar levels in people with diabetes by reducing insulin resistance.

Anti-inflammatory effects: The leaves contain compounds such as flavonoids and alkaloids that exhibit anti-inflammatory properties, which can help to reduce inflammation and pain.

Improving digestion: Pawpaw leaves contain enzymes such as papain and chymopapain, which aid digestion and can help alleviate digestive issues such as constipation and bloating.

It is important to note that while there is some evidence to support the medicinal benefits of pawpaw leaves, further research is needed to confirm these effects and determine appropriate dosages for use. Additionally, pawpaw leaves should not be used as a replacement for conventional medical treatment, and you should always consult with a healthcare professional before using any herbal remedies.

- Soursop leaves and Benefits.

Soursop is useful in fighting and preventing cancer. One study discovered that a soursop extract could shrink breast cancer tumors and kill cancer cells. A second study discovered that an extract could prevent leukemia cell formation. Flavonoids, phytosterols, and tannins are antioxidants found in the fruit and leaves of soursop, which have the inbred ability to fight cancer, amongst others.

**Nugget Three**

Get a couple of these leaves mentioned above together, (if you can get all of them, it will be better).  Rinse with clean water, boil them together and let it simmer for about 10 minutes then turn off the flame.

Allow the boiled mixture to steep or soak for about 10 minutes or until it is okay for you to drink,  however,  sieve out the water  and drink it warm.

All the same, you can take about one or two glasses of the sieved water. It is best to take it warm. Do these first things in the morning on an empty stomach and last thing at night.

Practice this routine continually. make it a lifestyle until healing changes are noticeable in your health conditions. It is also a remedy for so many common health challenges, for example feverish conditions, kidney issues, swollen limbs, high blood pressure and sugar levels and a general immune system booster.

**Nugget Four**

Get a couple of these leaves(do as previously mentioned in nugget three above), find a way to squeeze out the liquid out of them. Mix this liquid with fresh and pure palmwine, then take a glass or two first thing in the morning on an empty stomach and last thing at night.

**Note:** The quantity of each of the leaves should be virtually the same, starting with an amount you can consume within 48 hours without preservation.

Secondly, you can add more clean water to the squeezed out liquid, before mixing it with the palmwine on a 1:1 ratio. However, you can make the mixture to your preferred ratio.

Remember that it is not only pfor cancer problems. It can also boost your immune system against common and related health issues.

*Warning: Do not wait until you are ill before practicing these health nuggets in order to benefit from them, it is easier and better to prevent health issues than curing them. Start now!*

9 798378 207503